RELEASING CRANIAL/DURAL STRAINS,
ELIMINATING THE MYSTIQUE

RELEASING CRANIAL/DURAL STRAINS,
ELIMINATING THE MYSTIQUE

STEPHEN P. BRODERSON, DDS

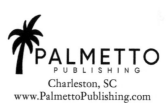

PALMETTO
PUBLISHING
Charleston, SC
www.PalmettoPublishing.com

Releasing Cranial/Dural Strains, Eliminating the Mystique

Copyright © 2021 by Stephen P. Broderson, DDS

First Edition

Paperback ISBN: 978-1-68515-447-9
eBook ISBN: 978-1-68515-448-6

ACKNOWLEDGMENTS

To my wife, Carole, who has been by my side as a counselor, lover, dental assistant, and best friend for over fifty-four years. She has made me who I am today.

To all my mentors and teachers, who have stimulated me to think independently and to realize my creative potential.

To my good friend and colleague Les Racowsky, DMD, for helping edit my manuscript. We spent many hours on the phone working together over the past six months.

Preface

The purpose of this book is to demonstrate to dentists and other whole-body practitioners a highly effective cranial release technique I have developed and refined over the past forty-five years. This release is a valuable adjunct for the treatment of head and neck pain and for the facilitation of movement of the teeth and bones when the dentist is treating dental orthopedic/orthodontic problems. As the reader gains experience with this technique, they will realize how dynamic the cranial/sacral system is. I hope that treating patients with the following techniques will open up an unending journey of awe and wonder with life and life energy.

Sometime during my first five years of practice, I observed changes in my patient occlusions that were treated to centric occlusion (CO) coincident with centric relation (CR). After some time, the mandible repositioned anteriorly and inferiorly, creating a "discrepancy" from CR to CO. If I adjusted the occlusion back to the coincidence of CR/CO, it would reposition again after some time. Several prominent practitioners were also experiencing these phenomena in their patients. I had X-ray documentation of the temporomandibular joint (TMJ) of these patients which showed no internal changes. Yet, the occlusion was changing. I concluded that there must be changes in the cranial vault bones, especially the temporal bones.

This experience led me to expand my knowledge by studying cranial osteopathy with Viola Frymann, DO, and applied cranial kinesiology with David Walther, DC. I also acquired three disarticulated human skulls in order to better examine the effects of what I had witnessed in my patients. I studied the individual bones and their sutures, the dura mater attachments on the inside, and the muscle/fascia attachments on the outside of the cranial vault. From these studies, I developed the cranial release technique demonstrated in the following book. The basic principle of the release is that if there is one area in the vault/face that is "strained" out of position, the whole cranium is affected, and the whole cranium must, therefore, be treated to get the system in harmony again.

Some of my more profound experiences with this technique are as follows:

- The first time I treated a patient with the release, I experienced an incredible increase in the amplitude and balance of the cranial rhythm. To this day, almost all releases result in a balanced rhythm with an increase in the amplitude.

- Early in the development of the release, I had a patient come in with a "bite that was only on one side," following an auto accident a month before. After treating him with the release, the patient could get his teeth together immediately on both sides!

- Many times in the early development of this technique, and continuing today, the release relieves a headache.

- I have treated many women at a local clinic I have worked at, who had pain related to chronic trauma from their spouses or significant others. The release has been very effective in relieving the pain related to this abuse.

- Recently, I treated a patient who had lost her husband and was experiencing severe anxiety, with head and neck pain, and on palpation, there was no movement. Also, there were involuntary spasms of the upper cervical muscles. After three treatments with the release, her anxiety and pain were resolved, the involuntary spasms reduced considerably, and she had normal cranial rhythm. She said to me the last time I saw her, "Thank you, Dr. Broderson. You have helped me so much."

Many of my patients have told me that the cranial treatment I utilize is the most profound they have ever felt, and they often ask to come back for more. For the past thirteen years, my wife and I worked two Fridays a month at a local clinic in our area treating pain dysfunction patients.. We had one patient that scheduled an appointment every time I was there for the past ten years, just to experience my "hands on work". He had allergies, and the release helped him to breath and sleep better after each treatment.

Releasing Cranial/Dural Strains, Eliminating the Mystique
A simple, concise, new technique

STEPHEN P. BRODERSON, DDS

HOW AND WHY TO USE THIS MANUAL.

The following cranial release techniques being presented are intended for use in conjunction with removable soldered lightwire orthopedic/orthodontic appliances. The combination of the releases with these appliances is a very effective treatment regimen for a pain dysfunction patient. Also these releases can be highly effective in preventing cranial pain after dental appointments, especially oral surgery, endodontics, and long restorative appointments where the patient has held his or her mouth open. Osteopathic literature is full of examples of patients with pain after oral surgery. Dental treatment is stressful for the patient and the dentist, needles for anesthesia, loud noises from the dental hand piece, poking around the teeth and gums with sharp objects, and rubber dam for some procedures making it impossible to get the mouth closed. For oral surgery, extractions can pull hard on the head and neck. All the work is in the mouth, close to the soul. The cranial release regimen presented in this book is highly effective for the dentist and the patient to relax at the end of an appointment. In most cases, the releases can be completed in fifteen minutes. Osteopathic cranial treatments balance the autonomic nervous system, improve the quality of sleep, and shorten the latency period for falling to sleep.

Other full-body practitioners may find this system very effective for their clients/patients. These regimens do not replace the need for ancillary help by an osteopath, chiropractor, or physical therapist. A review of the skull and the individual bones and dural membranes is recommended for readers. Both *Grant's Atlas of Anatomy* or *Gray's Anatomy* have excellent chapters showing the individual bones and the sutures.

Introduction

No cranial bone moves independently. Restrictions originating in
any part of the cranium will cause changes in the entire cranium.

—HAROLD IVES MAGOUN, *OSTEOPATHY IN THE
CRANIAL FIELD*

Not only do the cranial bones move, but they also move in a regular pe-
riodic cycle, which is often referred to as *primary respiration* or *cranial
rhythmic impulse* (henceforth referred to as CRI). This cycle circulates the
cerebrospinal/lymphatic fluid throughout the nervous system and the body.
The cycle has an inspiration phase, referred to as flexion, and an expiration
phase, referred to as extension. The cyclic CRI is independent of the pulmo-
nary respiration but can be affected by it. The average cycle occurs three to
ten times per minute and can be felt on the cranial vault as well as throughout the body. For CRI to occur, the cranial bones must move in concert with
other structures in what must be a flexible cranium, and thus they themselves
must be physically resilient and exhibit plasticity. Their movements are aug-
mented and controlled by the nature of the reciprocal tension membrane
(RTM) on the inside of the vault/sacrum and on the outside of the vault by
the nature and location of the muscle and fascial attachments on the outside
of the vault (see diagram below of the RTM).

In a normally functioning physiological cranial mechanism, the RTM controls the movement pattern (CRI), which can be palpated on the outside

of the cranium and on other parts of the body. For more information on cranial biomechanics refer to Appendix A. The RTM has strategic attachments to the inside of the cranium at the sutures and to other places on the cranial bones. For the movement pattern to be normal, there must be plastic resiliency within the bones themselves as well as at the sutures. Harold Ives Magoun, in his book, *Osteopathy in the Cranial Field,* further explains plastic resiliency of the cranium as necessary for the health of the system.

PLASTIC RESILIENCY

Every bone must be sufficiently resilient in itself and mobile at the sutures to move through its normal range of motion.

Contiguous bones must be similarly resilient and mobile to accompany movement or to compensate for movement without strain.

Dural membranes must be unrestricted in their areas of reciprocal tension to allow such movement to occur within normal limits. (Magoun, 1976)

The sutures are an integral part of the plastic resiliency of the cranial vault and face, they are actually joints with blood vessels, nerves, fibrous tissue, periosteum, and dura mater. The sutures of the vault are designed to allow for flexion(expansion) and extension (relaxation) during the cycles of the CRI. Interference with this normal physiologic movement (CRI) can result in a cranial strain. Magoun defines a cranial strain as "any alteration in cranial structure, sutural relations, or mechanical function resulting from a force within or without the body" (Magoun 1976).

A cranial strain leads to a distortion in the normal RTM which subsequently causes a distortion of the cranial vault and the maxilla. This can extend throughout the whole body. Cranial strains can result from either physical or mental trauma. A dental malocclusion can be a primary cause of a cranial strain because the tentorium cerebelli has attachments at the superior borders of the petrous apices of the temporal bones and is contiguous with the falx cerebri at the straight sinus. The mandibular condyles (temporal mandibular joint) articulate with the temporal bones bilaterally. Consequently, there is a direct structural relationship between the occlusion/mandibular position and the cervical vertebrae and sacrum. The following photo shows the cranial bowl from the superior view with the petrous apices of the temporal bones indicated with black lines. See Figures 1.1, 1.2, 1.3, and 1.4.

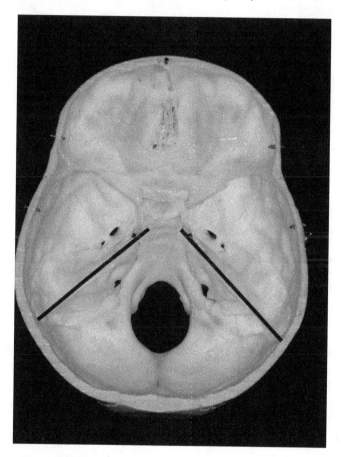

Figure 1.1 The black lines indicate the petrous apices of the temporal bones where the tentorium cerebelli have strategic attachments. Changes in the position of the temporal bones can directly effect the RTM.

The next photo shows a paper/wire model of the RTM in place over the temporal bones and the anterior portion of the cranial bowl.

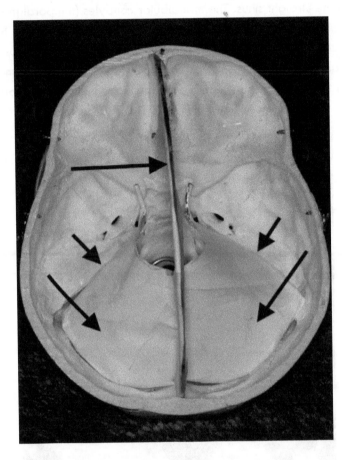

Figure 1.2 The upper arrow indicates the falx cerebri, the lower arrows indicate the tentorium cerebelli and the short arrows indicate where the tentorium cerebelli attaches to the temporal bones at the petrous apices. The superior border of the tentorium cerebelli connects with the falx cerebri in the midline at the straight sinus. These membranes make up the RTM in the cranial cavity. Refer to the photo below from Attlee's *Cranial Sacral Integration*, for an oblique view.

When cranial strains are present, they interfere with a person's ability to achieve optimal health by compromising the natural ebb and flow of the cerebrospinal and lymphatic fluid systems. The following figures show the RTM in the cranial cavity, and in the sacrum. In the release techniques described later the bones of the vault and face on the outside are used as handles to effect the RTM on the inside.

RECIPROCAL TENSION MEMBRANE

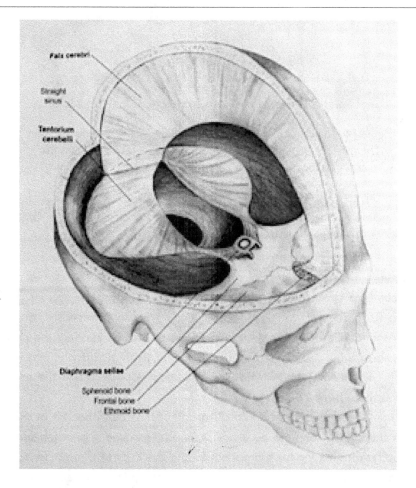

Figure 1.3 Intracranial dural membranes from *Cranial Sacral Integration* [Atlee 2012]. These membranes are the superior part of the RTM. The tentorium cerebelli has attachments to the petrous apices of the temporal bones. See above photos.

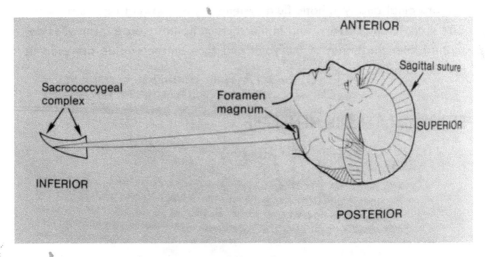

Figure 1.4 The above diagram shows the RTM, and is reproduced from *Craniosacral Therapy* [Upledger 1983]. Cranial dural membranes are contiguous with the upper cervical vertebrae and the sacrum.

As illustrated in the four previous figures, the dural membranes are part of a system that impacts the whole body. The bones of the cranial vault are lined with dural membranes. These membranes are contiguous with the periosteum through the cranial sutures on the outside of the cranial vault. They continue down the spinal cord and attach inside the sacrum, forming the RTM. The falx cerebri, falx cerebelli, tentorium cerebelli, and the diaphragma sellae are folds in the dura mater that extend into the cranial cavity, separating the parts of the brain. With strategic attachments inside the vault, foramen magnum, and upper cervical vertebrae and the sacrum, they constitute the RTM.

Chronic tension can result in a distortion of the vault because of the nature of the RTM. When the dura are strained ("torqued"), or when some of the muscles attached to the cranial bones and are in chronic spasm (e.g., from occlusal stress), the sutures of the vault can become immobilized ("jammed," "stuck"). This immobility results in changes in the flow of cerebrospinal fluid. As John Upledger suggests, "When the dural membranes are subjected to tension in a certain direction over time, the fibers in the membrane tend to organize in the direction of the tension" (Upledger 1983). This is why correcting a dural strain can be long term in a grown patient. Permanent asymmetries in the bones of the cranial vault and face can result from a long term strain originating in birth or child hood.

Muscle Attachments

Skeletal muscles attach to the periosteum on the outside of the skull and mandible and cross the vault sutures (e.g., masseter, temporalis, and sternocleidomastoid). Cranial strains can result when muscle activity is imbalanced or excessive. This is because the periosteum on the outside of the skull is contiguous through the sutures with the dural membranes on the inside of the skull. Anterior and posterior cervical muscle attachments can have similar adverse effects upon dural balance.

The occlusion, which ultimately controls the mandibular position in all three-dimensions, is extremely important for optimal function of the cranial sacral system. Treating the mandibular position is an integral part of releasing a strained cranial system because the origins or attachments of the muscles responsible for mastication cross over the critical sutures of the sphenoid, temporals, frontal, occiput, and parietals. Fascial attachments from the mandibular periosteum to the periosteum on the outside and base of the skull exist primarily through the sphenomandibular and stylomandibular ligaments. Posterior cervical muscles originate at the occiput, and some, like the splenius capitis and the longissimus capitis, cross the *occipitomastoid suture* (OMS). The sternocleidomastoid originates across the OMS and inserts into the sternum and clavicle. The hyoid musculature, in combination with the intrinsic muscles of the tongue, are also important for the balancing of the system through their attachments to the temporals, the sphenoid, the occiput, and the hyoid bone. The three-dimensional position of the mandible affects the functional length of these muscles.

Technique Basics

You may consider the bones of the cranial vault simply as hard places in the dural membranes.

—UPLEDGER, *CRANIOSACRAL THERAPY*

The understanding of these techniques is based upon the understanding of the range of motion of the vault and facial bones in all three dimensions. If one or more of the bones of the vault or face are "strained or locked," *the entire system* is adversely affected. The overall release of the system occurs through implementing a combination of the individual releases that follow. An individual bone's range of motion is determined by several factors, including its suture designs, the nature of the attachments of the dura to the interior of the vault, and the muscle attachments to the periosteum on the outside of the vault. As a result, there will be variations in range from patient to patient.

Ultimately, release occurs because the body seeks equilibrium. When the bones of the vault/face are carried through their range of motion, determined by suture design, traction is *applied indirectly* to the dura. A back-and-forth motion within each bone's range of motion and within its flexibility releases the dural strain indirectly.

A useful analogy for how this release occurs would be a balloon stuck in a twisted position. To release the twist, one would hold the balloon and then exaggerate the twist by applying gentle pressure in the direction of the twist then backing out of the twist. By going in and out several times until the twist releases, it allows the balloon to return to normal without the risk of being damaged.

Before beginning the actual release regimen on a patient, monitor the CRI for balance, frequency, and amplitude. Remarks should be made in the record for comparison after the release has been performed.

- Balance: Are movement and character [strong/weak] equal on both sides of the vault?

- Frequency: How long is the cycle? How many cycles per minute?

- Amplitude: How strong, weak, oscillating?

Palpation in this context is the therapist attempting to feel the CRI. It is performed by placing the forearms and hands alongside the patient's head while they are lying supine or at an angle in the dental chair. The palms of the hands should be opposite the parietal bulges, with the fingers over the mastoid processes of the temporal bones, and the thumbs resting lightly over the lateral vault portions of the frontal bone. See Figures 2.1 and 2.2 The rest of the therapist's body should be relaxed and comfortable with both feet on the floor and their mind blank. It is crucial to have a *very light touch*. For some, it is easier to feel the CRI with the hands and fingers slightly away from the head (see the photos below). When palpating for the CRI, wait for a cycle to come, it may come on the flexion or extension part of the cycle, it may not be present at all, or just on one side, or it may feel like it is moving diagonally across the vault, or it may move in an anterior to posterior direction. All of these variations are the result of the mental or physical trauma the patient has experienced. I have experienced a rolling of the energy from the left side to the right on several patients that were beaten on the left side by a right-handed person. For me, the CRI is more a feeling of energy, than physical movement. Following the complete release regimen, palpate the CRI again and record any changes that have occurred.

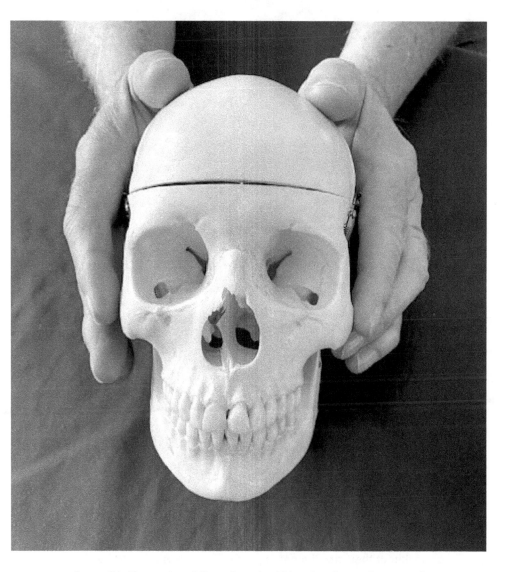

Figure 2.1 The center of the palms should be placed over the parietal bulges. This is where the CRI can be felt most easily.

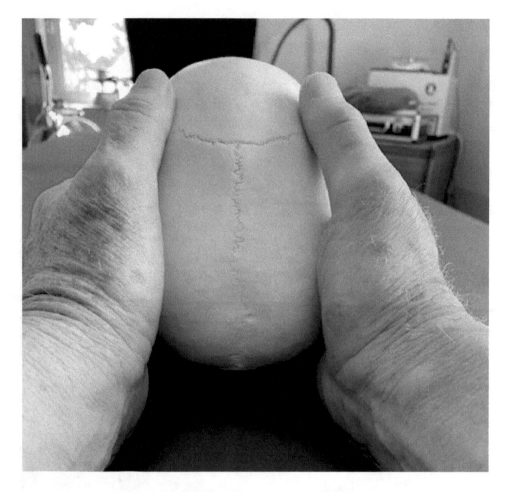

Figure 2.2. It is most important to have a very light
touch when attempting to feel the CRI.

Patients undergoing dental orthopedic treatment should be palpated both
with and without their appliances in place. The release should be done after
the appliance has been adjusted and is in place as it will then be possible
to know what effect the appliances and their adjustments have on the CRI.

The following is a description of palpating the CRI, as experienced by
Thomas Attlee DO, from his book *Cranial Sacral Integration*

When palpating CRI ...our touch so soft and light that we are barely touching the head, we can observe even with our hands off the body, we can still feel these movements, qualities and asymmetries. What we are picking up is the movement of a universal force which pervades all the tissues of the body but which extends beyond the tissues...we are engaging with the matrix.

This matrix is present in early embryonic life, forming an energy field...which is present as a force field within which we exist, visible to some as aura, palpable to some as a cushion or field of energy. What we are feeling when we palpate the CRI is a combination of structural mechanical movement and inherent life energy. We are tuning into is not specifically bones, membranes, or fluids, but to the subtle energy or vitality through these structures and beyond these structures, the movement of the whole energy matrix which incorporates the bones, membranes and fluids, but which does not specifically consist of them. (Atlee 2012)

My interpretation of what Dr. Attlee states in the above, is the CRI is more energy movement than physical bone fascia movement, controlled by the matrix, which is the origin of life energy itself.

Releases are performed by facilitating (rather than by forcing) and directing the bones into their physiologic position within the primary respiratory system and allowing the body to return to its normal rhythm. The therapist should regard the bones as "hard places within the dural membranes" (Upledger 1983). All forces used in the releases should be one pound or less. I recommend the reader go to the supermarket and place a finger on a vegetable scale and press down until one pound is registered. You will realize how little a pound of force is.

Techniques in Detail

ANTERIOR CRANIAL RELEASE

The zygoma/frontal lift is the first move in the release of the vault. The *frontal* articulates with the sphenoid and both parietals, both zygomata and maxillae on the outside, the ethmoid within the vault, and both nasal and lachrymal bones within the orbit.

The anterior attachment of the falx cerebri is at the crista galli of the ethmoid, (see photos of the RTM model) and the superior sagittal sinus is in the anterior superior portion of the frontal bone, so the falx may be manipulated indirectly by moving the frontal bone in a horizontal and horizontal-lateral direction. The coronal suture, the frontal sphenoid suture, and the frontal ethmoid suture are all oriented in the horizontal plane.

The frontal is released in an anterior direction, parallel with the Frankfort horizontal plane. The frontal lift is done in conjunction with and to facilitate the zygoma release and the maxilla release.

Sutures of each zygoma are on the outside of the frontal, sphenoid, maxilla, and temporal bones. The zygomata can be considered capstones to the cranial vault and face, so they are released first. The zygomata connect the anterior cranium with the posterior cranium bilaterally on the outside of the vault at the temporal zygomatic sutures.

The zygoma forms the lateral and part of the inferior borders of the orbit and articulates outside the vault with the maxilla, the temporal, and the frontal bones. Within the orbit, the zygoma articulates with the greater wing of the sphenoid.

Together with the maxilla and the temporal, the zygoma forms the zygomatic arch, which provides the origin of the masseter muscle. In bruxism and clenching, this muscle can lock up the zygomatic temporal suture, preventing motion in the whole vault. The zygomatic arch provides room for the coronoid process of the mandible in opening and in lateral movements.

The zygoma is released in an anterolateral direction, approximately thirty to forty-five degrees from the midsagittal plane. The zygoma has a vertical axis of rotation that runs from the zygomatic frontal suture down through the posterior portion of the zygomatic maxillary suture.

Upledger reminds us to "consider the bones of the cranium simply as hard places in the dural membranes" (Upledger 1983). Patient comfort and safety is key, so ensuring a light touch is important. All releasing forces should be kept at approximately one pound or less.

After the CRI is assessed, the frontal is grasped behind the orbital processes with one hand, placing a thumb on one side and a forefinger or middle finger on the other. With the opposite hand, the tip of the little finger or forefinger is placed under the zygomatic arch on one side as far anterior as is possible. Please refer to [Figures 3.1 and 3.2] for a demonstration of this hand placement. Traction of the frontal is done in the anterior (horizontal) direction. As this is being done, the zygomatic arch is gently (using less than one pound of force) lifted in an anterolateral direction, about thirty to forty-five degrees to the midsagittal plane.

On the side of the zygoma release, the frontal should first be moved straight forward then rotated to the side opposite the zygoma being released. The zygoma release is held until some "softening" is felt for three to five seconds. After this, the other side should be is addressed, and the other zygoma released in the same manner. Several back-and-forth movements may need to be performed before both zygomatic arches are "softened" (released).

In the following photos, Figures 3.1 shows the right zygoma lift on the skull, Figure 3.2 shows the right zygoma lift on the patient, Figure 3.3 shows the left zygoma release on the skull, and Figure 3.4 shows the left zygoma release on the patient. The photos demonstrate the finger and hand positions for the zygoma/frontal release.

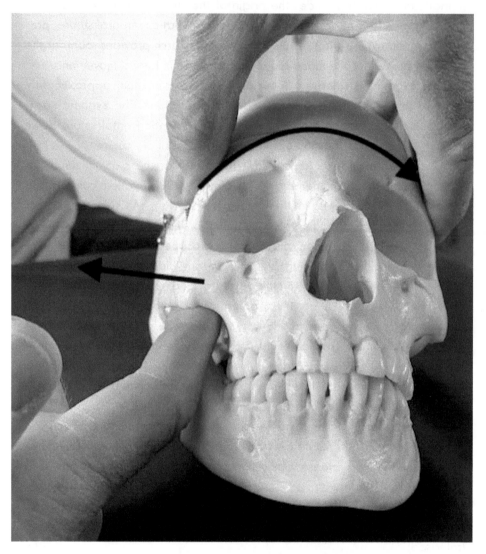

Figure 3.1 Right zygoma release. The frontal is lifted and rotated in the horizontal plane while the zygoma is lifted away at thirty to forty-five degrees from the midsagittal plane.

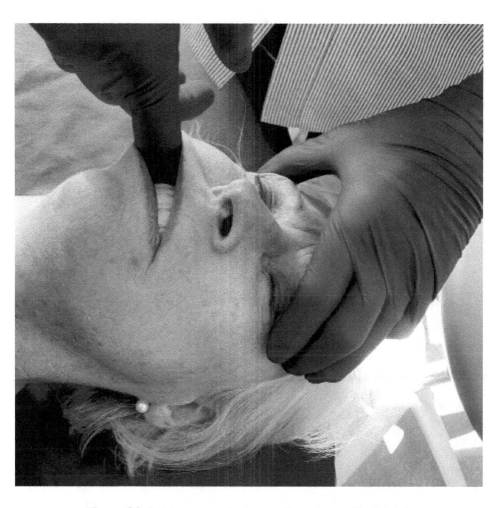

Figure 3.2 Right zygoma release on a live patient. The frontal
is lifted and rotated to the left while the right zygoma is lifted
thirty to forty five degrees from the midsagittal plane.

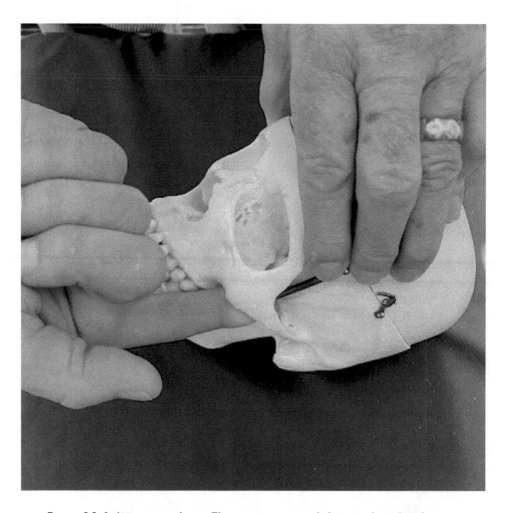

Figure 3.3 Left zygoma release. The zygoma is moved thirty to forty-five degrees anterior in the horizontal plane, while the frontal is lifted and rotated to the right.

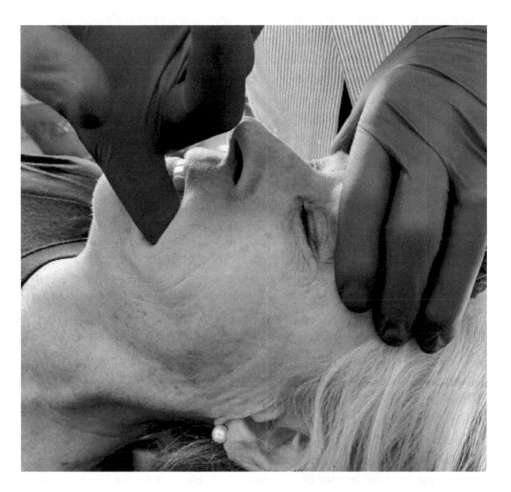

Figure 3.4 Left zygoma release on a live patient.

Since the RTM is under constant tension, this combined move increases the tension on the falx cerebri, releasing the coronal suture, the frontal, the sphenoid, and the ethmoid, and begins to release the temporals. Sometimes, in cases of long-term dysfunction, there will be difficulty getting the zygoma to release, so you may have to treat several times. These patients will often be the clencher/bruxers. It is common to have one side very restricted, which may cause the release to be somewhat painful. After the release occurs, the pain will be greatly reduced. This usually occurs on the internally-rotated side. Many times, I have experienced an increase in the amplitude of the CRI from the zygoma/frontal lift.

MAXILLA RELEASE

The maxillae articulate with each other and the vomer at the midpalatal suture, the palatines posteriorly, with each lamina orbitalis of the ethmoid superior, and with the frontal in the midline, forming each side of the bridge of the nose. The maxillae also articulate with the lachrymals and nasals within the orbit and laterally with the zygomata.

The palatine maxilla articulation (the cruciate suture) releases in a horizontal anterior-posterior direction parallel with the palate. The sphenoid is indirectly affected through the palatine sphenoid and the cruciate sutures. Thus, each maxilla can become a handle for engaging the sphenoid indirectly.

The maxillae release that occurs in the superior/inferior (vertical) direction at the anterior border of the sphenoid is allowed by the bilateral articulation of the medial pterygoid plates where they engage the grooves in the pyramidal processes of each palatine. The sphenovomerine suture in the midline (the articulation of the vomer with the rostrum of the sphenoid) also allows rotation of the maxillae in the sagittal plane.

An internal maxillary rotation on the *right* side can be released externally by holding the anterior portion of the maxilla with the right thumb over the labial root surfaces of the central and lateral incisors, while the first and second fingers are placed on the palate opposite the first and second molars. The right maxilla is held with the thumb as a pivot point anterior, and the posterior portion is pushed laterally and slightly posterior with the two fingers, along a path visualizing the angles of the lateral pterygoid plate. For the *left* internally rotated maxilla, the first two fingers of the same hand are placed over the labial root surfaces of the left central and lateral, the thumb is placed on the lingual of the palate opposite the first and second molars, and the fingers become the pivot point while the thumb pushes the posterior maxillary buccal slightly posterior, again along the angle of the pterygoid plates.

The maxillary internal rotation releases described above work best in combination with a removable, soldered lightwire appliance that can be adjusted unilaterally to create a force to correct an internally rotated side of a maxilla.

MAXILLA/FRONTAL/ETHMOID/SPHENOID RELEASE

This release utilizes the frontal and maxilla as "handles" *to indirectly* release the ethmoid and the sphenoid. Again, the frontal is grasped behind the orbital processes with a thumb on one side and the forefinger or middle finger of one hand and held in light *horizontal* traction. The maxillae are held with the thumb and forefingers of the other hand on each side at the upper second molars, and the maxillae are pulled gently first in an *anterior* direction and then rotated to one side while the frontal, under traction and with less than one pound of force, is rotated in the opposite direction. See Figures 4.1 and 4.2. It is very common to feel the maxillary rotation restricted towards one side or the other. This indicates a sphenoid restriction on the side of the restricted maxillary rotation.

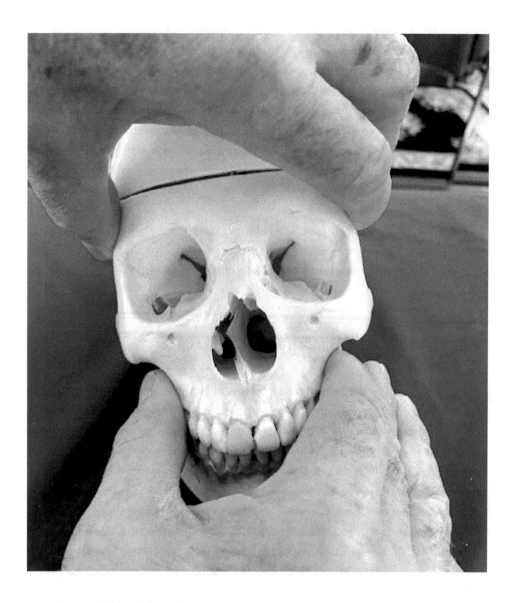

Figure 4.1 Maxilla/frontal counter rotation occurs in the horizontal plane. Both the maxillae and the frontal are gently pulled anteriorly in the horizontal plane and then counter rotated. The rotations are reversed several times.

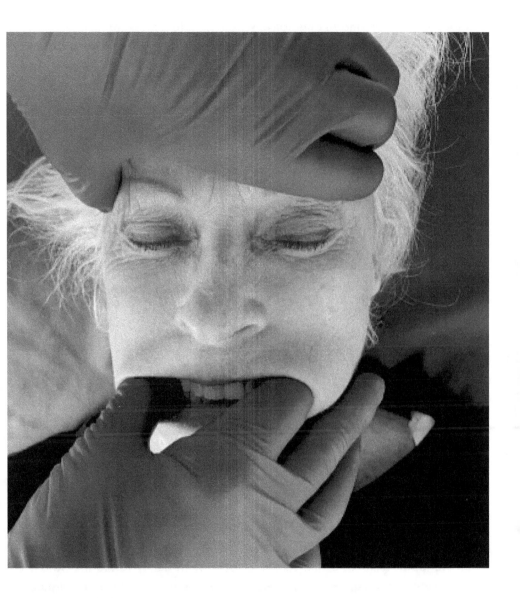

Figure 4.2 The frontal is lifted and rotated in one direction while the maxillae are rotated in the opposite direction. Then the movements are reversed.

These releases are made alternatively from right to left several times before progressively including an anterior and inferior release, first on one side then on the other. On one side, as the frontal is lifted and stabilized and with a slight anterior superior movement on that side, the maxilla is tipped inferior while it is pulled anterior, creating a vertical decompression of the cranium on that side. The other side is then pulled down and anterior while the frontal is tipped slightly superior, decompressing the cranium on the other side. This movement is similar to a sidebend.

Anterior traction on the maxillae with rotation on the horizontal plane decompresses the sphenosquamous suture (temporal) and the sphenoid frontal on the side opposite the maxillary rotation. This also compresses on the side of the rotation. This back-and-forth motion of the maxillae, rotation with traction, helps release the above named sutures. When you first engage the maxilla with anterior traction and rotation you are feeling the most anterior portion of the RTM, the falx cerebri. Many times it will feel rigid all the way to the upper cervical vertebrae. As you counter rotate the frontal with the maxillae several times there will be a release and the rotation will become less restricted. For all releases, focus, visualize the sutures and the dura, and use your intuition to follow the system. You are engaging the life force of the patient.

Flexion and extension movements affect the maxillae, frontal, and ethmoid at their common sutures. It is also possible to use these releases to bring these bones into flexion and into extension. As part of the complete release regimen, movement of the maxilla into flexion and extension will help the practitioner to feel where the system is restricted. See Figures 5.1, 5.2, 5.3, and 5.4. To bring the maxilla into flexion, a finger is placed on the midpalatal suture at the anterior flat portion of the palate with the thumb placed on the labial surfaces of the central incisors. Then gently rotate the palate superiorly and anteriorly, visualizing the change at the sphenoid palatine and sphenoid vomer areas.

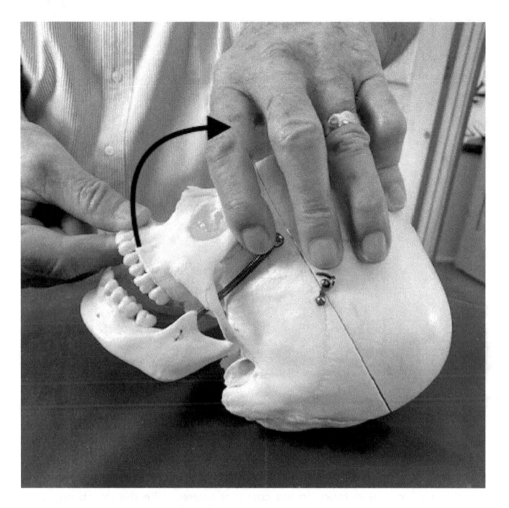

Figure 5.1 Maxilla is brought into flexion with a superior anterior pull on the anterior portion of the maxillae.

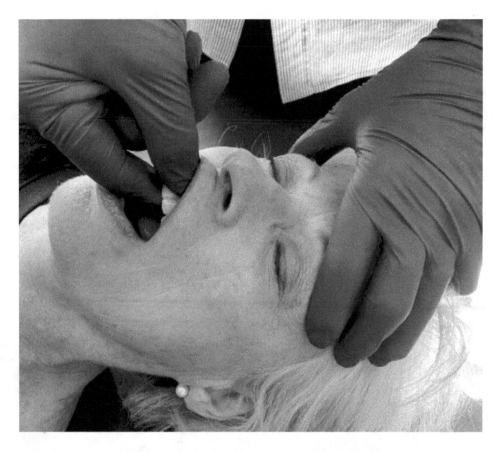

Figure 5.2 Maxilla into flexion on a live patient

To then bring the maxilla into extension, the finger is moved more posteriorly in the midline, just anterior to the cruciate) suture. With the thumb on the same place on the central incisors, gently rotate the posterior of the palate superiorly while bringing the incisors inferiorly. As you are doing these moves you will be able to feel which phase of the CRI is restricted. Record your findings in the record so you can tell on subsequent visits if the restriction has changed.

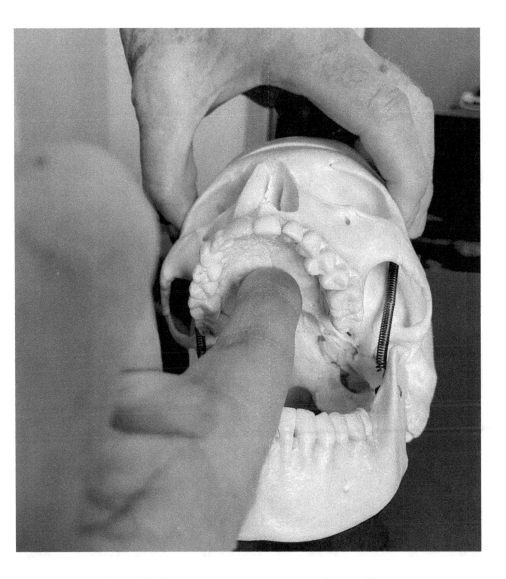

Figure 5.3 Finger position for extension of the maxilla, in
the midline, just anterior to the cruciate suture.

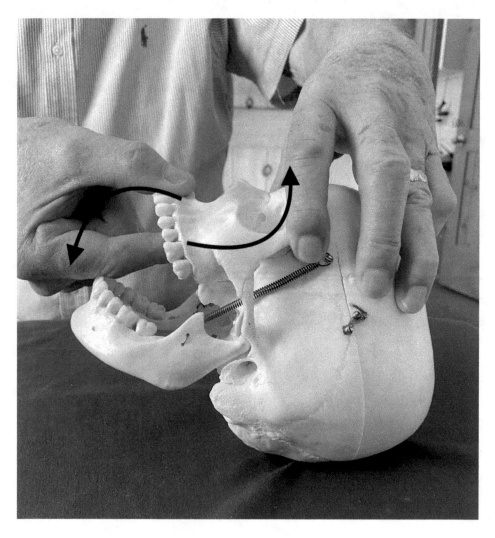

Figure 5.4 Thumb and finger positions to bring the maxilla into
extension. The posterior maxilla is rotated superiorly and posteriorly,
while the anterior is pulled inferiorly and posteriorly.

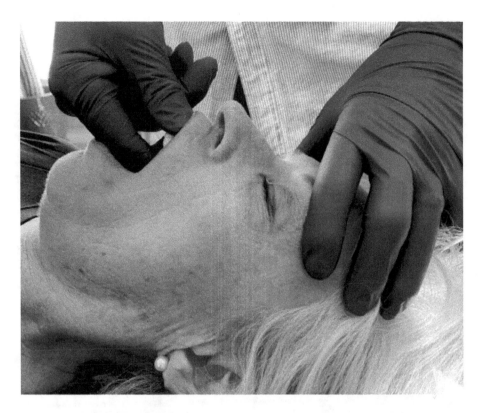

Figure 5.5 Maxilla into extension. During these two moves, it is possible to feel the positional change of the maxilla relative to the sphenoid.

ETHMOID/FRONTAL RELEASE

While holding the frontal in horizontal traction as described earlier, place the finger and thumb of the other hand on either side of the lachrymal/nasal/frontal processes of the maxillae, just slightly into both orbits. The frontal processes of the maxillae can then be moved first to one side and then the other several times in a horizontal and lateral direction until equal softness is felt left and right. See Figures 6.1 and 6.2. This releases the anterior portion of the falx cerebri at the crista galli of the ethmoid and the ethmoid itself in the midline.

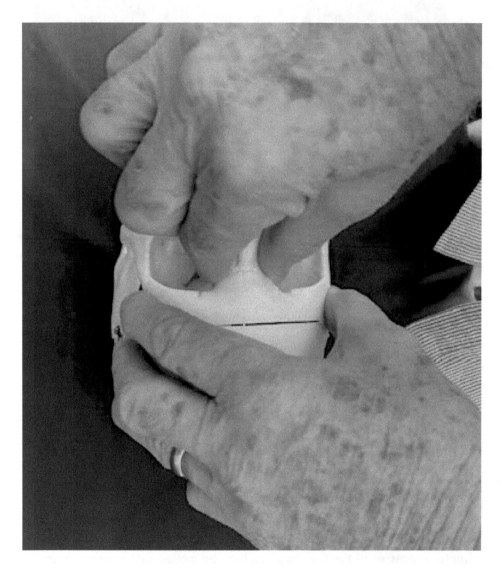

Figure 6.1 The ethmoid "slides" from right to left horizontally against the frontal until it feels equal on both sides. This is very effective for releasing congested sinuses.

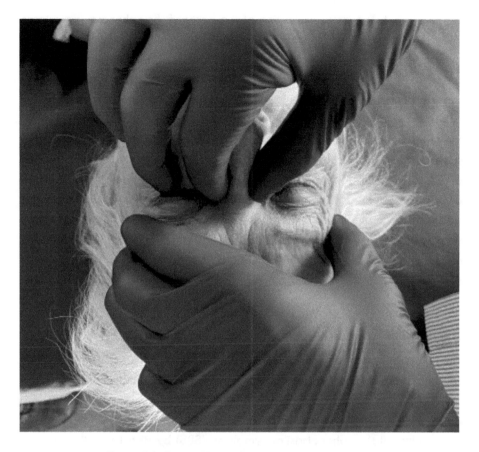

Figure 6.2 Ethmoid/frontal release on a live patient.

POSTERIOR CRANIAL RELEASES

Sphenoid

The sphenoid is released indirectly by the zygoma/frontal lift, maxilla frontal counter rotation, flexion and extension of the maxilla, the ethmoid frontal release, internal and external rotation of the temporals, and manipulation

31

of the occiput. The anterior portion of the body of the sphenoid articulates with the ethmoid, and the vomer in the midline. Anterior laterally the greater wings articulate with the zygomata, and the parietals, and inferior at the pterygoid plates with the palatines . The posterior portion of the sphenoid body articulates with the occiput in the midline. The lateral and posterior of the greater wings articulate with the temporal bones. During flexion of the temporal bones the squama move lateral, and the petrous apices move superior. The gear train action of the sphenosquamous suture and the rise of the SBS tips the sphenoid anterior towards flexion. A dental occlusion can affect the sphenoid through the palatines and the vomer, especially if the posterior vertical dimension is altered. Dural attachments at the anterior and posterior clinoid processes of the sphenoid permit traction of the dura mater when the positions of the sphenoid, the maxillae, and the temporals are changed.

The Mandible

The mandible with the dental occlusion is an integral part of the cranial sacral system. For the dentist this is especially important, because changes in the occlusion can affect cranial balance.

Mandibular traction places an anterior and inferior force on the base of the cranium at the sphenobasilar symphysis (SBS) by distracting the suspensory ligaments, the sphenomandibular ligaments, and the stylomandibular ligaments. Traction on these ligaments produces movement similar to the extension phase of the primary respiratory cycle.

See Figures 7.1, 7.2, 7.3, and 7.4. The mandible can be distracted, or pulled inferiorly and anteriorly by placing the thumb of one hand on the occlusal surface of the lower second molar and the fingers of the same hand under the anterior of the body of the mandible. While using the other hand to stabilize the cranium with a frontal hold, gently rotate the mandible anterior and inferior while pulling the anterior portion of the mandible superiorly and anteriorly. Hold and wait for four to five seconds until softening occurs. Switching hands, repeat this process on the other side. It will be necessary to go back and forth until both sides feel released. One side may feel much more restricted than the other, indicating a sphenoid or temporal problem on that side, and may have to be treated several more times to get equal release.

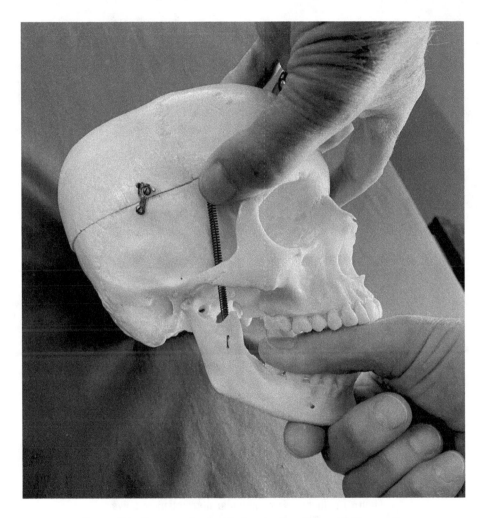

Figure 7.1 Downward anterior traction on the mandible results
in pulling the base of the cranium toward extension.

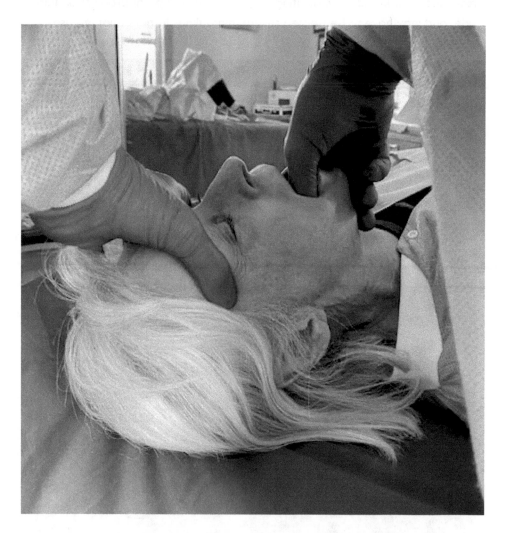

Figure 7.2 Right side mandibular distraction on a live
patient. The force is downward and anterior.

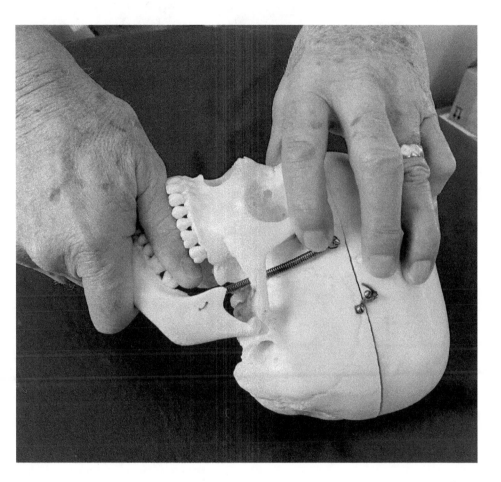

Figure 7.3 This is the same movement on the left side. Many times one side
will be more restricted than the other, indicating sphenoid restrictions.

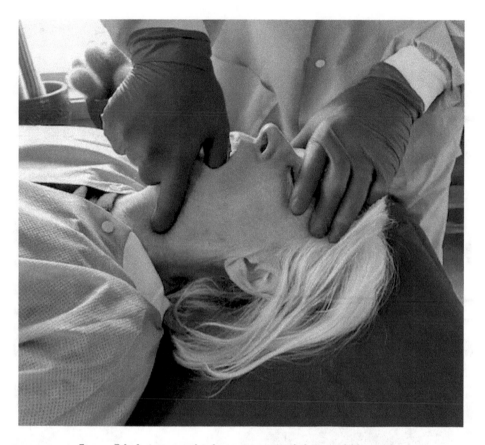

Figure 7.4 Anterior and inferior traction of the mandible can be
used to apply an extension force to the cranial base.

Temporals

The temporal bones articulate with the sphenoid, the occiput, the zygomata, and the parietals. The path of insertion of the temporals is anterior and horizontal, approximately forty-five degrees from the sagittal plane, and is parallel with the petrous portions relative to the occiput and the sphenoid. See Figures 1.1 and 1.2 above.

Dural attachments (tentorium cerebelli) at the apices of the petrous portions of the temporals allow for indirect traction on the falx cerebri. The temporal bones can be put into external rotation by moving the mastoid process posterior medial and into internal rotation by moving the mastoid process anterior lateral. The temporals have a gliding and rotational motion, rotating around the petrous apices while gliding along the OMS. This gliding motion occurs because the temporal bone also has a horizontal axis of rotation. This horizontal axis goes from the spheno-squamous pivot anteriorly through the most posterior portion of the temporal where it articulates with the occiput. On this axis, the temporal glides horizontally, anteriorly, and posteriorly while it pivots away from the occiput and sphenoid in the horizontal plane during flexion.

Moving the temporal bones into internal or external rotation results in a stretching of the tentorium cerebelli and a change in the falx cerebri. Magoun describes the following:

> *traction on the falx cerebri,.... changes the fluid pressure within the vault. Alternately rotating the left and right temporals into internal and then external rotation with these movements, you will feel a considerable amount of fluid motion, ultimately helping balance the system. Lateral fluctuation is common. A transverse wave may be deliberately initiated to bring the fluid to a state of equilibrium for that pattern to incite more activity when the fluctuation is weak or uneven. This is done by rotating the petrous portions of the temporals in the opposite directions simultaneously.* (Magoun 1976)

RELEASING THE TEMPORALS

The above quote was most influential in integrating the following temporal bone release into the overall release regimen presented in this book.

The right and left temporals are released simultaneously by moving one side into external rotation and the opposite side into internal rotation, then reversing the hands to move the temporals in the opposite directions. See Figures 8.1, 8.2, 8.3, 8.4, 8.5, and 8.6. These combined moves constitute the temporal bone release. To begin the release, place the palm of one hand under the occiput with the fingers extending toward the opposite side behind the cranium. Place the thumb on that hand anterior to the mastoid process on that side and the first and second fingers of the opposite hand posterior to the mastoid process of the other side. During the internal rotation force the second finger supports the first finger, while the first finger engages the posterior side of the mastoid process. Simultaneously, move the mastoid process with the thumb of the supporting hand posterior and medial(towards external rotation), while the first and second fingers of the opposite hand bring the mastoid on that side anterior and lateral(towards internal rotation). The angle of release may vary from patient to patient and from side to side—be aware and adapt. Remember, you are a facilitator. Do not force any movement; follow the system. Then the hands are reversed with the thumb anterior to the mastoid process on the other side, while the fingers of the other hand are posterior to the mastoid process of the opposite side. See the photos of the hand placement on the skull. See Figures 8.1 and 8.4.

The mastoid processes are used to move the temporal bones in opposite directions *simultaneously*, creating a torquing of the dura (tentorium cerebelli and falx cerebri) and the SBS. The hands are reversed and the temporals are moved simultaneously on the opposite side. In my experience, the temporal bone release has the most influence for allowing an increase of the amplitude of the CRI.

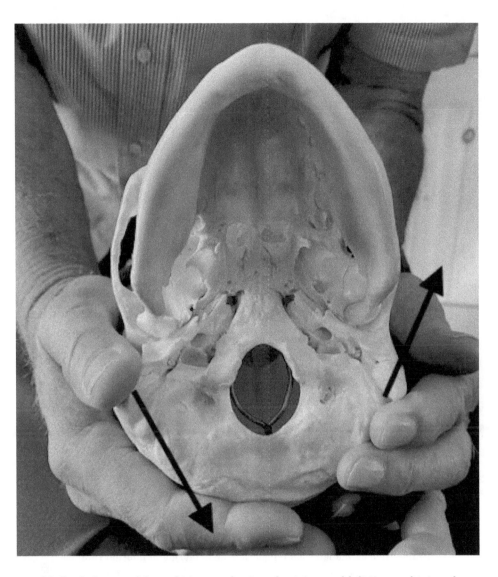

8.1 Hand placement for right temporal external rotation and left temporal internal rotation Arrows indicate the direction of the forces applied simultaneously. They are nearly perpendicular to the petrous portions of the temporal bones, posterior medial on the external rotation side and anterior lateral on the internal rotation side.

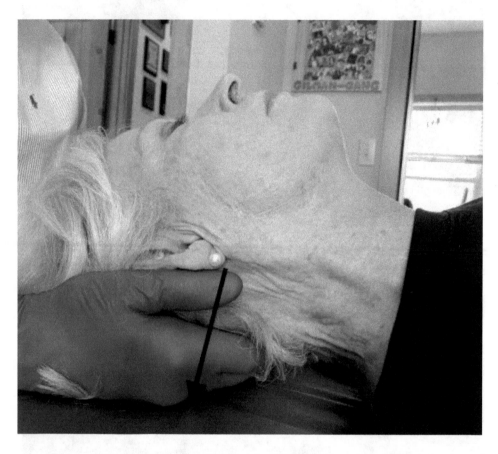

Figure 8.2 Right side temporal external rotation on a live patient. The right thumb is anterior to the mastoid process and moving it posterior-medially at the same time as the left side temporal bone is moving in internal rotation.

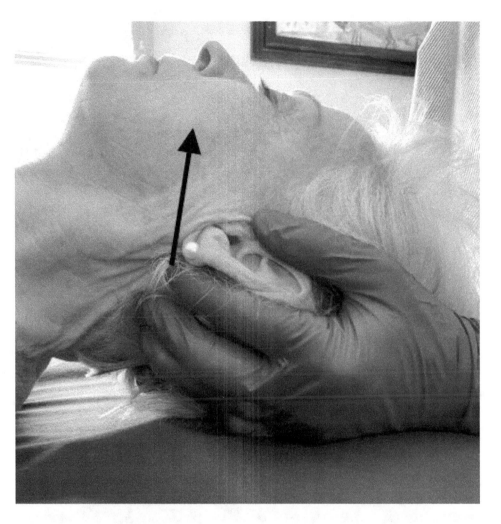

Figure 8.3 Left side temporal internal rotation on a live patient.
The first and second fingers of the left hand are posterior to
the mastoid process, moving it anterior-laterally.

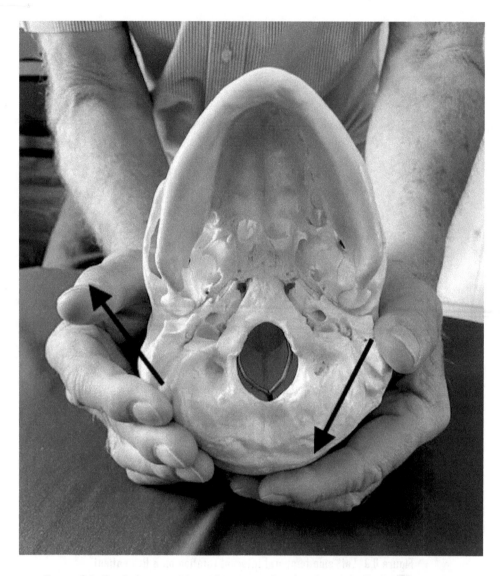

Figure 8.4 Hand placement for right temporal internal rotation, and left temporal external rotation.. The hands are reversed with the left thumb anterior to the left mastoid process, and the right fingers posterior to the right mastoid process, moving the temporals internal rotation right and external rotation left, simultaneously

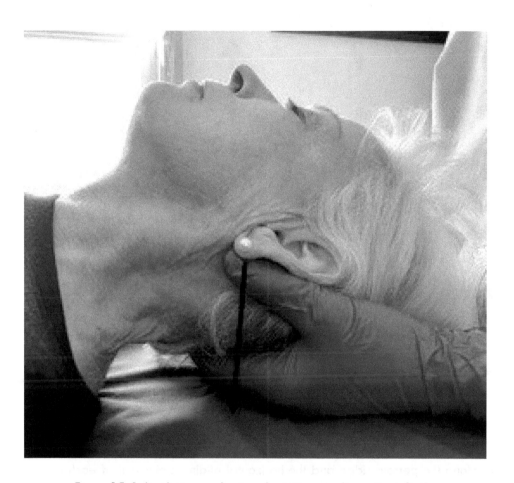

Figure 8.5 Left side temporal external rotation on a live patient. On the patient, the left thumb is anterior to the left mastoid process, moving it toward external rotation, while the right first and second fingers are posterior to the mastoid process moving it toward internal rotation.

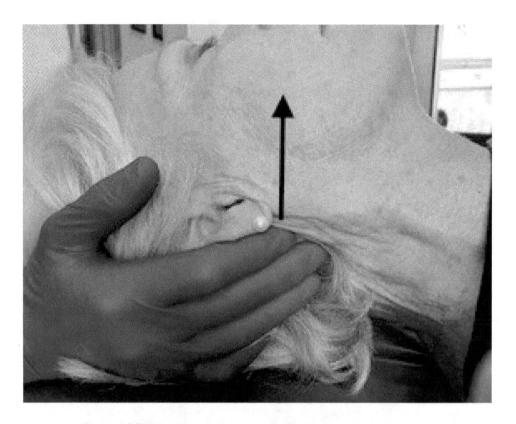

Figure 8.6 Right side temporal internal rotation on a live patient. The
right first and second fingers are posterior to the right mastoid process,
moving it toward internal rotation. The arrow points up.

It is important not to force this motion, but rather to feel the axis of rotation
along the petrous ridge and the horizontal gliding movement of each temporal bone. No more than one pound of force should be used.

Often, patients with strains will have a restriction on one or both sides,
and repeated treatment may be necessary to obtain a balanced system.
Each "side cycle" should take three to four seconds then be followed by a
one- to two-second pause, and lastly a reversal to the other side for another
three to four seconds. Several repetitions may be necessary to achieve balance and equal movements. The mastoid processes should be as symmetrical as possible at the finish.

OCCIPUT

The occiput has articulations with the sphenoid at the SBS, the temporals, the parietals, and the atlas/axis (vertebral column). The occiput is indirectly affected through the temporal bones, the sphenoid, and the atlas/axis in the upper cervical spine. The SBS has flexibility, even after union at around age sixteen. In this area, flexion and extension originate, resulting in internal/external rotation of the paired bones.

The occiput has circumferential dural attachments at the foramen magnum and continues up to the falx cerebri via the falx cerebelli. The tentorium cerebelli is attached to the falx cerebelli at the straight sinus in the center, lateral-horizontally via the transverse sinuses, and anterior along the petrous apices of the temporal bones, with ending attachments at the posterior clinoid processes. See Figure 1.2.

The occiput can be indirectly affected through manipulation of the temporal bones or directly affected through contact at the external occipital protuberance. The sternocleidomastoid muscle and the splenius capitis muscle both originate across the OMS. Therefore, a spasm in either of these two muscles can cause jamming or restriction at the OMS.

UPPER THREE CERVICAL VERTEBRAE

The spine is connected to the occipital bone at the atlanto-occipital joint at the occipital condyles. These joints are condyloid synovial joints. Below the dural attachment at the foramen magnum, the cervical attachments of the dura mater are at the first, second, and third vertebrae through the anterior and posterior longitudinal ligaments and the myodural bridge at the second cervical vertebra (C2). The tentorium cerebelli is directly connected to the upper cervical vertebrae by extension of the dura mater through the foramen magnum into the upper cervical vertebrae. Thus, malocclusions also often have cervical problems.

Traction of the dural cervical spinal attachments is done by holding the base of the cranium at the occiput with two fingers of each hand and pulling in the superior direction along the plane of the spine while gently rotating the vault alternately to the right and left. See Figures 9.1, 9.2, 9.3, and 9.4.

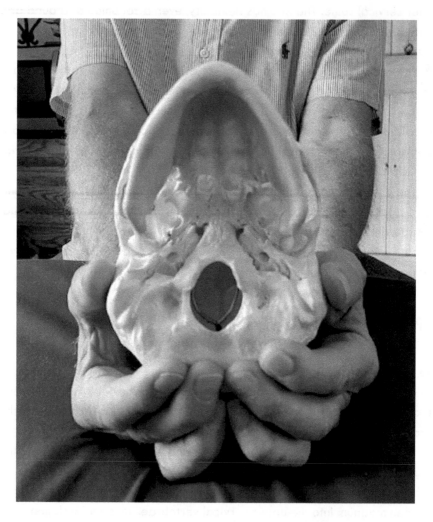

Figure 9.1 Upper Cervical vertebrae release. The first and second fingers of each hand grasp the base of the occiput as far under the skull as possible and traction in a superior direction. This is most effective if done while the CRI cycle is in extension.

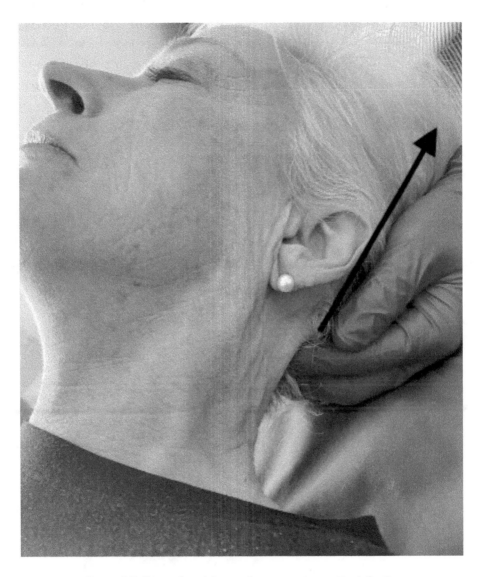

Figure 9.2 Cervical vertebrae release on a live patient. On the patient, the fingers of both hands grasp the base of the occiput as far under as possible and traction in a superior direction.

To aid in the release of the atlas occiput and atlas and axis vertebrae, hold the base of the occiput with one hand, utilizing gentle superior traction. Then, alternately move the spinous processes of the second and third cervical vertebrae (C2 and C3) with the middle fingers of the other hand several times, first to the left then to the right. The C2 is usually the most prominent superior spinous process.

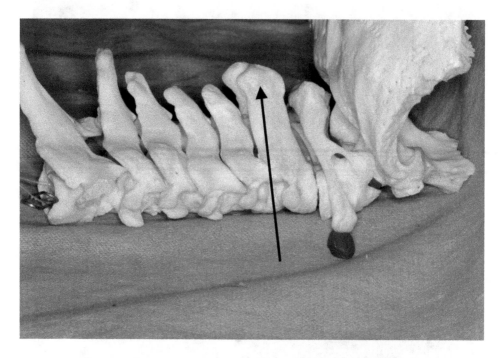

Figure 9.3 Lateral view of the occiput with cervical vertebrae. The arrow points to C2 spinous process, easily felt on most patients.

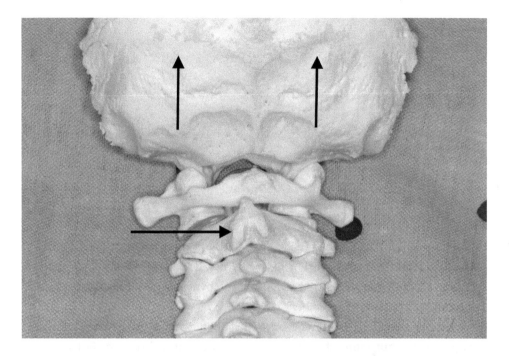

Figure 9.4 The fingers of one hand traction the occiput superior while the other hand's fingers move C2 to one side then the other.

Tenderness, restriction, or displacement may be encountered in one direction or the other and indicates rotation of the vertebrae. To address this, move down the cervical spine and move C4 through C6 to the right and left. The origin of the semispinalis capitis is just below the superior nuchal line, bilaterally near the midline, and inserts into the lateral border of the transverse processes of C3 through the third thoracic vertebra (T3).It is common for it to be tender to palpation.

These releases should be followed once again with the temporal release to ensure unrestricted temporal bone movement.

Completion and Dismissal

Completion of these releases should include an assessment of the CRI. The CRI is sometimes disrupted (paused) by the above cranial manipulations. Osteopaths refer to this as the "still point." Movement may take from a few seconds to a minute to resume.

Usually there will be an increase in amplitude, the frequency of which may change, but there should be an improvement in balance. Balance is best assessed by feeling even amplitude of the cranial motion on both sides. When the CRI is balanced, the mastoid processes of the temporal bones will usually feel more symmetrical.

Correction of CRI Imbalance

If there is an imbalance in the CRI, one mastoid may be in internal rotation while the other is in external rotation. Palpate the rhythm, and when the system goes into the extension phase, the internally rotated side can be released by rotating it externally (placing the thumb anterior to the mastoid, then gently rotating in a posterior and inferior direction), while the externally rotated side is held neutral.

When there is a cervical displacement to one side, the spinous process of C2, C3, or both can be gently moved toward the midline. This release should also be made during the extension phase, and the release repeated for three cycles.

It is very common to observe a combined displacement of the cervical vertebrae and the temporal bones. This can be treated by releasing the internally-rotated temporal externally while gently assisting the spinous process toward the midline again for three cycles of extension. Again, begin the release when the system transitions into the extension phase, and continue the release through three phases of extension of the CRI.

The efficacy of treatment can best be determined by assessment of the CRI. The assessment should be made before treatment and compared with the assessment made after treatment. Assessment can also be done utilizing applied kinesiology before and after the release. See Appendix B for detailed explanation of Applied Kinesiology. Muscle test with therapy localization at the following points: sagittal suture, occipital-mastoid suture, and the center of the sacrum. Test both with the teeth together and with the mouth wide open. If there is weakness with the teeth together, the occlusion is causing the weakness. If the weakness occurs with the mouth wide open, there is a cranial problem. Record these results, then after the release, do the muscle test again. There should be a strong test at a previously weak suture point if the release has been effective. Muscles in spasm may also be utilized for assessment of treatment for the posterior cervicals, sternocleido-mastoid, and masseters. The sternocleidomastoids are particularly sensitive to temporal bone position.

These releases can be to be used by a dental practitioner after any appointment lasting more than thirty minutes as merely holding one's mouth open for extended periods can cause locking up of the cranial system. Crown preparations, hygiene care, extractions (especially), periodontal sur-gery, and any other procedure where a rubber dam is used can subvert the cranial rhythm. In real-time circumstances, the total cranial release should take approximately ten to fifteen minutes, with chronic pain patients taking up to thirty minutes.

Treatment with soldered wire appliances, other orthodontic/orthopedic appliances, or any appliances treating the dental occlusion should be moni-tored with assessment of the CRI. This should take place both with and with-out the activated appliances as well as before and after adjustment.

It is important to note that this system does not replace the need for ancillary help (osteopathy, chiropractic, or physical therapy) because many whole-body problems are associated with cranial mandibular dysfunction.

References

Attlee, Thomas. 2012. *Cranio-Sacral Integration*. London: Singing Dragon.

Brinker, Thomas et al. 2014. "A new look at cerebrospinal fluid circulation." *Fluids and Barriers of the CNS* 11:10

Enix, Dennis E. DC, et al. 2014. "The cervical myodural bridge, a review of the literature and clinical implications." *The Journal of the Canadian Chiropractic Association* 58, no. 2 (June): 184–92.

Gehin, Alain. 1985. *Atlas of Manipulative Techniques for the Cranium & Face*. Seattle: Eastland Press.

Jones, L. et al. 1982. "Significance of nerve fibers interconnecting cranial suture vasculature, the superior sagittal sinus, and the third ventricle." *Journal of the American Osteopathic Association* 82:113.

Magoun, Harold Ives. 1976. *Osteopathy in the Cranial Field*. 3rd ed. Indianapolis: The Sutherland Cranial Teaching Foundation, the Cranial Academy.

McPartland, J.M. and Mein E.A. 1997 "Entrainment and the cranial rhythmic impulse." Altern Ther Health Med. Jan;3(1): 40-5.

Nelson, Kenneth E. et al. 2006 "Recording the Rate of the Cranial Rhythmic Impulse" *Journal of the American Osteopathic Association* Volume 106, No 6

Retzlaff, Ernest W., and Frederic L. Mitchell, eds. 1987. *The Cranium and Its Sutures.* New York: Springer-Verlag Berlin Heidelberg.

Sampson, H. Wayne, John L. Montgomery, and Gary L. Henryson. 1991. *Atlas of the Human Skull.* Texas: Texas A&M University Press.

Upledger, John E., and Jon D. Vredevoogd. 1983. *Craniosacral Therapy.* Seattle: Eastland Press.

Walther, David S. 1981. *Applied Kinesiology Volume 1.* Systems DC, Pueblo, Colorado.

List of Figures

Figure 1.1 The cranial bowl with the petrous apices of the temporal bones indicated.

Figure 1.2 The cranial bowl with the tentorium cerebelli and the falx cerebri indicated.

Figure 1.3 Intracranial dural membranes, a diagram of the skull with the RTM (Atlee 2012).

Figure 1.4 The RTM of the whole body (Upledger 1983).

Figure 2.1 Anterior view of hand positions for CRI palpation.

Figure 2.2 Posterior view of hand positions for CRI palpation.

Figure 3.1 Right zygoma lift on the skull.

Figure 3.2 Right zygoma lift on a live patient.

Figure 3.3 Left zygoma lift on the skull.

Figure 3.4 Left zygoma lift on a live patient.

Figure 4.1 Maxilla frontal counterrotation on the skull.

Figure 4.2 Maxilla frontal counterrotation on a live patient.

Figure 5.1 Flexion of maxilla on the skull.

Figure 5.2 Flexion of maxilla on a live patient.

Figure 5.3 Finger placement for extension of maxilla.

Figure 5.4 Extension of maxilla on the skull.
Figure 5.5 Extension of maxilla on a live patient.

Figure 6.1 Ethmoid frontal release on the skull.
Figure 6.2 Ethmoid frontal release on a live patient.

Figure 7.1 Right side mandibular distraction on the skull.
Figure 7.2 Right side mandibular distraction on a live patient.
Figure 7.3 Left side mandibular distraction on the skull.
Figure 7.4 Left side mandibular distraction on a live patient.

Figure 8.1 Right thumb and left hand finger placement on the skull for right temporal external rotation and left temporal internal rotation.
Figure 8.2 Right thumb placement on a live patient for right temporal external rotation.
Figure 8.3 Left hand finger placement on a live patient for left temporal internal rotation.
Figure 8.4 Left thumb and right hand finger placement on the skull for left temporal external rotation and right temporal internal rotation.
Figure 8.5 Left thumb placement on a live patient for left temporal external rotation.
Figure 8.6 Right hand finger placement on a live patient for right temporal internal rotation.

Figure 9.1 Upper cervical vertebrae release on cervical bones.
Figure 9.2 Cervical vertebrae release on a live patient.
Figure 9.3 Lateral view of cervical vertebrae and occiput bones.
Figure 9.4 Posterior view of cervical vertebrae and occiput bones with arrows to show direction of release forces.

Appendix A

CRANIAL BIOMECHANICS

The craniosacral system is composed of the dural membranes, the individual movements of the cranial bones themselves at their sutures, the muscles in and around the head and neck, the circulation of the cerebrospinal fluid/lymphatic/circulatory system, and the neural proprioceptive system that controls the body's homeostasis. The mandible with the occlusion of upper and lower teeth and the accessory ligaments of the temporomandibular joints are also an integral part of the craniosacral system.

Magoun, in his book titled *Osteopathy in the Cranial Field*, describes the two phases of the rhythm of the craniosacral system: *flexion* (inspiration) and *extension* (expiration). Flexion and extension refer to the movement of the midline bones, which are the occiput, sphenoid, ethmoid, and vomer (see Figure 2). The remainder of the vault and facial bones (referred to as paired bones) move into *external rotation* during the flexion of the midline bones and *internal rotation* during the extension of the midline bones. Paired bones include the temporal bones, the zygomata, the maxillae, the palatines, and the nasal bones with the conchae. There is a bending at the sphenobasilar and sphenoethmoid areas of the cranial base.

As the system moves toward flexion, the occiput rotates counterclockwise from the right, the sphenoid rotates clockwise, the sphenobasilar area rises, and the ethmoid rotates counterclockwise (see Figure 2). As the occiput rotates counterclockwise, it causes the petrous portions of the temporals to rise and move anterolaterally, rotating clockwise. The temporals rotate about an axis that is oblique, along the petrous portions of the temporal, almost through the external auditory meatus. This rotation brings the mastoid process posteriorly and slightly medial (Magoun 1976). Because the glenoid fossa is anterior to the center of rotation of the temporal, it moves slightly inferior and posterior. Concurrently the anterior portion of the ethmoid is rotating up, bringing the anterior segment of the maxilla with it.

In the posterior maxilla, the articulation of the palatines with the pterygoid plates of the sphenoid causes the posterior portion of the maxillae to move inferiorly and widen (Magoun 1976). The combined movement of the temporal fossae/condyles and the posterior portion of the maxilla inferior during flexion and superior during extension allows the posterior teeth to contact during each phase of the cycle. In flexion, the temporal fossae/condyles move inferiorly and posteriorly, a CL II tendency. In extension, the opposite occurs; the temporal fossae/condyles move anteriorly and slightly superior, toward a CL III. In swallowing, the tongue places an anterior superior force into the maxilla (flexion). As the teeth come together with the muscle force vector in an anterior superior direction, the temporals and maxillae are moved toward extension. These opposing forces balance the cranium.

This motion is cyclic, occurring at the rate of three to ten times per minute. This rhythmic cycle can be altered by physical and mental trauma, leading to a locking of the sutures. One of the causes of this trauma is thought to be inadvertent orthodontic forces, leading to cranially caused chronic disorders.

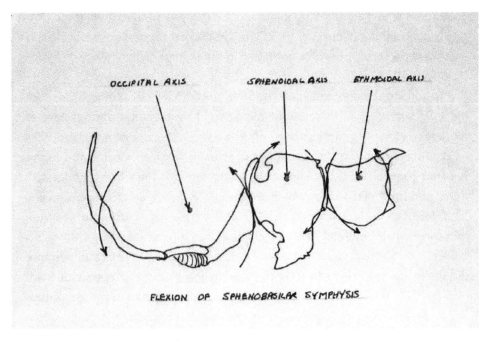

OCCIPITAL AXIS   SPHENOIDAL AXIS   ETHMOIDAL AXIS

FLEXION OF SPHENOBASILAR SYMPHYSIS

Figure 2. The occiput, sphenoid, and ethmoid viewed from the right side during flexion. The maxilla follows the ethmoid, and the temporal follows the occiput.

CEREBROSPINAL FLUID AND ITS CIRCULATION

The craniosacral system is characterized by rhythmic mobile activity that persists throughout life (Upledger 1983). It was thought to be a semiclosed hydraulic system, with the fluctuation of cerebrospinal fluid (CSF) production controlling the rhythm (Upledger 1983). As the CSF pressure increases, the cranial vault expands because of the unique design of the sutures. As early as 1982, an article described a neural control mechanism that shuts down the CSF production when it reaches a certain level, causing the rhythm that can be palpated on the outside of the cranium (Jones et al. 1982). More recently an article described a comparison of the Traube-Hering-Mayer oscillations with the cranial rhythmic impulse (CRI) and found them to be palpably concomitant (Nelson et al. 2001). Cranial osteopaths have developed treatment protocols based on normalizing the cranial rhythm (Magoun 1976; Upledger 1983).

Traditional osteopathic understanding of the CSF circulation states that the CSF originates in the choroid plexuses within the ventricular system of the brain; circulates through the ventricles, the cisterns, and the subarachnoid spaces; and is absorbed in the arachnoid bodies concentrated in the superior sagittal sinus. Choroid tissue is suspended in the CSF of the lateral, third, and fourth ventricles (Brinker et al. 2014). However, this recent review by Brinker et al. indicates that the CSF circulation is much more complex than previously believed. The CSF circulation comprises not only a directed flow of the CSF but also a pulsatile back-and-forth movement throughout the entire brain with fluid exchange among the blood, the interstitial fluid, and the CSF. This is possibly what is felt when the cranial rhythm is palpated. There is a continuous bidirectional flow of fluid exchange at the blood-brain barrier, which exceeds the CSF production rate by far. The CSF circulation around the blood vessels of the Virchow-Robin spaces provides for major drainage as well as a clearance pathway for the waste molecules from the brain as well as interaction of the systemic immune system with the brain (Brinker et al. 2014).

ORIGIN OF THE CRANIAL RHYTHMIC IMPULSE

The ultimate cause of the CRI is not fully understood, but it seems the concept of entrainment is most likely to encompass this issue. Entrainment is the integration or harmonization of oscillators. These oscillators include cardiac pulse and heart rate variability, Traube-Hering modulation, diaphragmatic excursion, contractile lymphatic vessels, CSF production by the choroid plexus, pulsating glial cells, electrical fields generated by cortical neurons, cortical oxidative metabolism, and probably many other oscillators. All organisms pulsate with a myriad of electrical and mechanical rhythms

(McPartland and Mein 1997). The CRI is the palpable perception of entrainment because of a combination of several body rhythms incorporated with the individual practitioner's own rhythms. For a successful outcome of a treatment session to occur, the practitioner must have a balanced autonomic system with a calm demeanor. In a successful therapeutic process, the patient's and therapist's systems entrain (Attlee 2012). When this occurs, the patient's own rhythms are subconsciously invited to join with the practitioner as the session progresses, and good outcomes will result.

Appendix B

APPLIED KINESIOLOGY AND CRANIOMANDIBULAR DYSFUNCTION MONITORING HUMAN BIOENERGY—MUSCLE PROPRIOCEPTORS

A pplied kinesiology was developed in the early sixties by George Goodheart Jr., DC. Based on the work of Kendall and Kendall in the 1930s, *Principles of Manual Muscle Testing*, Goodheart found that muscle testing could be used to find weaknesses in the body's structural, chemical, and mental systems. He called this the triad of health, with structure at the base of the triangle and chemical and mental at the other sides of the equilateral triangle. With outward changes in each of these entities, muscle testing could be used to find and verify corrective means to return the body to health.

Goodheart found "the body heals itself in a sure, sensible, practical and observable manner. 'The healer within' can be approached from without. Man possesses a potential of recovery through the innate intelligence or the physiological homeostasis of the human structure. This recovery potential for which he is endowed merely awaits for the hand and the heart and the mind of a trained individual to bring it into manifestation allowing health to come forth; this is man's natural heritage" (Walther 1981).

Muscle testing requires knowledge of the individual muscle's origin and insertion and bracing techniques to allow the muscle being tested to be isolated (not recruited by other muscles). This is important for getting accurate information. Recruiting of other muscles can lead to an ambiguous result.

In the treatment of craniomandibular dysfunction, muscle testing can be invaluable in finding the problem, the source of the problem, and most important, the way to treat the problem. Muscle testing can also be used to validate the treatment. All muscle testing should be done with the patient standing. The practitioner *must* be completely neutral when utilizing muscle testing, as the results can be influenced by mental attitudes. You are looking for information about the patient's energy system—bioenergy.

Muscle testing, in combination with *therapy localization* (see no. 2 below), is a way of finding information about the body that cannot be acquired in any other way. The following demonstrates the technique:

1. With the patient standing, find a muscle that tests strong by itself (in the clear). For our needs, the deltoid is the best muscle. For right-handed people, stabilize the right shoulder of the patient with your left hand. Then have the patient hold their left arm out straight with the elbow locked out and the palm down. Place the first two/three fingers of your right hand over the patient's forearm just above the wrist and apply downward pressure for one to one and a half seconds. You are attempting to find the muscle's resistance to stress. Repeat this one to two more times so you feel/remember the resistance of the muscle. It is easy to overpower the muscle.

2. Therapy localization (TL) is touching an area that you suspect may have a problem. For craniomandibular disorders, touch the TMJ joints just in front of the ear, the occipital mastoid suture (OMS) on both sides, the spinous processes of the upper cervical vertebrae, and the center of the sacrum. The patient will touch one of these points with the first two fingers of the other hand, with the remaining fingers folded under the thumb. Then the strong muscle will be tested to find a difference in the muscle response. If there is weakness in the indicator muscle, there is an energy disturbance in the area

being therapy localized. The test does not tell you what the cause of the disturbance is, only that there is one. If the muscle tests strong with TL, then there may not be an energy problem in that area.

3. Challenge: Asking the body what the cause of the energy disturbance is or what the treatment could be. For example, TL the right and left TMJ and test the indicator muscle (IM). The muscle tests strong. Test again (challenge) with the teeth together, and if the IM weakens, you know the closed position is causing the muscle to weaken. You do not know why. You can challenge the position by changing the mandibular position (by placing cotton applicators between the upper and lower first molars). If the IM tests strong, there is a posterior vertical deficiency.

4. Sometimes the vertical needs to be higher than the cotton applicators, then utilize the May swallowing reflex, especially in denture wearers. Use prosthetic rope wax, make two pieces double thickness about one-half to three-fourths inch long, and place them in warm water. Then on each side, place the wax over the occlusal surfaces of the lower molars and the second bicuspids, and squeeze the wax vertically to open the bite. Place your hands gently on the patient's shoulders, and tell the patient to rest on the pillows and then slowly close and swallow. They are *not to go through the wax* so that their teeth contact. Do this four to five times, each time pressing the wax up vertically, and when you observe consistent consecutive easy swallows, measure the interincisal opening at the upper/lower incisors with the teeth resting on the wax. This is the swallowing reflex vertical. Record this measurement. Muscle test again while the patient rests on the wax, TL the TMJ joints and the suture points that you previously tested, and you will find the muscle will respond with much more strength. Now you know that there is deficient posterior vertical support.

AREAS TO EXAMINE VIA TL

The areas to examine via TL are cranial sutures at occipital mastoid bilaterally, the sagittal suture, bregma, lambda, and nasion. Based on the author's experience, the OMS is highly sensitive to a poor occlusal position. Also test with TL at the ends of the spinous processes of the upper cervical vertebrae and the center of the sacrum. Test each TL point with the teeth together and also with the mouth wide open. With the mouth wide open, weakness indicates a cranial problem at that TL point, not associated with the mandibular position. Weakness at the sutures with the teeth together indicates an associated occlusal/cranial problem. Weakness in closed and open position indicates cranial and occlusal problems. Challenge the system by changing the mandible position and test again (cotton tip applicators or swallowing reflex). You may find that changing the mandibular position will correct both the closed and the open mouth weakness, indicating the occlusal position is the cause. It is common to see a relationship between the mandibular position and problems in the cervical vertebrae.

OTHER TESTS UTILIZING TL

A test for over coupling of the anterior teeth is done by having the patient touch a finger to the outside of the upper anterior teeth with the teeth together. Weakness indicates over coupling of the anterior teeth. Then have the patient pull the upper anterior teeth forward for five to ten seconds and test again. A strong test supports the hypothesis that the anterior teeth are over coupled.

Physiologic orthodontic/orthopedic appliance adjustments can be verified by therapy localizing the sutures before and after the adjustment. This should include verifying the vertical dimension of a TMJ/cranial appliance (the May pivot appliance).

Also prosthetic devices crossing the maxillary midline can be tested to determine if they are causing cranial problems. It is common for a fixed bridge crossing the midline to "lock up" the cranial mechanism. Therapy localize the bridge as well as the nasion, OMS, and cervical vertebrae with the mouth open and closed.

There is vast information to be gained utilizing applied kinesiology in your practice. It is a way to gain information from your patients that no other modality can give. Remember to be completely objective.

Muscle proprioceptors (spindle cells) monitor muscle length and are concentrated in the belly of a muscle. The closing muscles have vast numbers of spindle cells. The opening muscles have few or none. According to literature, the lateral pterygoid has 4–6, the masseters have 114, and the temporalis have 342 (Kubota and Masegi 1977).

Golgi tendon organs (GTOs) monitor tension and are active in reflex regulation during normal function. GTOs are found in the muscle/tendinous attachments of the muscles.

The above proprioceptors can be manipulated to change the muscle response, that is, the muscle can be "turned up" or "turned down."

If a muscle is found to be weak "in the clear," it can be turned up by doing the following:

1. Activate the muscle spindle, that is, traction the midbelly toward the origin and insertion of the muscle, several times and retest. The muscle will respond with strength.

2. Activate the GTO at the origin and insertion by pressing toward the center of the muscle.

3. The opposite can be done to the spindle cells and the GTO to turn down a muscle.

This technique can be used for chronic muscle spasms of the masseters, temporalis, and posterior cervical muscles, that is, the trapezius. When one side is in spasm, turn up the opposite side and turn down the overactive side (Walther 1981).